# ISSUES IN
# HUMAN SEXUALITY

A Statement by the House of Bishops
of the General Synod of the Church of England,
December 1991

CHURCH HOUSE PUBLISHING
Church House, Great Smith Street, London SW1P 3NZ

**ISBN 0 7151 3745 X**
GS Misc. 382
Published 1991 for the General Synod of the Church of England
by Church House Publishing

*John Bates*
*Richard Harries*
*Bill Russan*
*(Paul Lucas)*

*Rowan W.*
*roypher.*

Printed in England by Tasprint

# Table of Contents
## by Chapter and Paragraph

2. contd.

5. contd.

# Preface

The 1988 Lambeth Conference called on all bishops of the Anglican Communion to undertake in the next decade a 'deep and dispassionate study of the question of homosexuality' (Resolution 64). This Statement from the House of Bishops is partly a response to that call as well as being our reflection on the pastoral situation we face in our own Church and society. In formulating it we have been greatly helped by the work of a small group, chaired by the Bishop of Salisbury. We have also been assisted by the opportunity to share these issues and this Statement with all our brother bishops in the Church of England, including those who are not members of this House.

Our purpose has been 'to promote an educational process as a result of which Christians may both become more informed about and understanding of certain human realities, and also enter more deeply into the wisdom of their inheritance of faith in this field' (para. 1.9).

We cannot expect all to agree with our conclusions and, indeed, in our own discussions we encountered a wide variety of opinions and we benefited by vigorous debate, set as it was in the context of mutual affection and tolerance. It is our hope that this Statement – which we do not pretend to be the last word on the subject – will do 'something to help forward a general process, marked by greater trust and openness, of Christian reflection on the subject of human sexuality' (para. 1.9). We encourage clergy chapters and congregations to find time for prayerful study and reflection on the issues we have addressed.

On behalf of the House of Bishops

+ GEORGE CANTUAR
*Chairman*

*November* 1991

# 1. Introduction

1.1    As Bishops of the Church of England we are conscious of the anguish of spirit felt by many members of our Church today over the issue of homosexuality. There is the pain and anger of those who grieve over changes in the sexual morality of our society, and who feel that the Church does not respond with a sufficiently clear scriptural and traditional word and witness. There is the pain and anger of gay and lesbian people who feel rejected by both past and present attitudes among Christians, and also of heterosexual Christians who are distressed by these attitudes and penitent for them. As chief pastors we ourselves know the pain of being torn between the conflicting demands of individuals and congregations, of particular ministers and the Church's ministry as a whole, of the integrity of faith and morals and the dignity to be accorded to all men and women, made in God's image. In what follows we have tried, as those entrusted with guarding Christ's truth and caring for his people, to be faithful to what we have been shown of his mind.

1.2    These are questions in which deep levels of the personality, feelings and fears often unconscious or unexamined, come into play, affecting the way each person thinks and argues, speaks and behaves. The same applies to the effects of cultural environment and conditioning. Such factors will plainly have had their influence on what we say here, just as they will on the way it is received. It can therefore be no more than one stage in a discussion which needs to be continued throughout the Church by individuals and groups who learn humbly and prayerfully to be open to facts, to one another, and to Scripture, Tradition and reasoned reflection on experience. Only so shall we discover how the word of the Gospel is to be made living flesh in our day, and how all of us are to grow in the power of the Spirit into a greater maturity in which 'mercy and truth are met together, righteousness and peace have kissed each other'.

1.3    Theologically there is a particular reason why these questions could hardly be more sensitive, namely that they arise from some of the sharpest controversies of faith in the Church at this time. They concern the way Scripture and Tradition are to be understood, and the authority which these are to have in matters of human living. How are we to approach the biblical witness to God's self-revelation in order to discern the divine will for ourselves today? What are the consequences for scriptural interpretation of critical scholarship or new scientific

1

knowledge or new sensitivities arising from changing experience? These are matters which in principle and in general terms have been examined for us over recent years in the Church of England in such publications as *Christian Believing* (1976), *Believing in the Church* (1981), *The Nature of Christian Belief* (1985) and *We Believe in God* (1987). But specific issues present particular difficulties.

1.4    On the major issue with which we are here concerned a landmark for the Church of England in recent years was the report *Homosexual Relationships,* published for the General Synod Board for Social Responsibility in 1979. This consisted in the main of a document from a Working Party chaired by the Bishop of Gloucester (the so-called 'Gloucester Report'), to which were added 21 'Critical Observations' by the Board itself. Taken as a whole this was a major contribution to discussion within the Church of England, but because of the controversy it aroused it perhaps failed to promote as much serious debate as might have been hoped for. In 1989 another BSR Working Party produced a further substantial and valuable document (the 'Osborne Report') to guide and assist the thinking of the House of Bishops, which had indeed commissioned it. Because of the status of this text the House refused permission for its publication, though a copy did make its way unofficially into the possession of the media. We wish to put on record here our gratitude for the help this Report has given us, not least through its faithful attention to what homosexual people themselves have to say, and through the openness and respect for people which mark its style and approach. What is striking, however, as one reads both Reports, is how little the main lines of argument have changed in the ten years that separate them. Details have changed – on some scientific points, on biblical exegesis, and in the volume of testimony from homosexual people themselves – but of any substantial agreement there seems as yet little sign.

1.5    It is important to recognise that in facing this situation the Church of England is not alone. The 1988 Lambeth Conference revealed deeply-felt divisions within the Anglican Communion in this area, and the Report, *The Truth Shall Make You Free,* has this to say in the section 'Christianity and Social Order', under the heading 'Sexual Orientation':

> We recognise that this issue remains unresolved, and we welcome the fact that study is continuing. We believe that the Church should therefore give active encouragement to biological, genetic and psychological research, and

consider these scientific studies as they contribute to our understanding of the subject in the light of Scripture. Further study is also needed of the socio-cultural factors which contribute to the differing attitudes towards homosexuality ... in the various Provinces of our Church. We continue to encourage dialogue with, and pastoral concern for, persons of homosexual orientation within the Family of Christ (paras. 154–155).

The passage quoted then refers to Resolution 64, which begins as follows:

This Conference:
1    Reaffirms the statement of the Lambeth Conference of 1978 on homosexuality, recognising the need in the next decade for 'deep and dispassionate study of the question of homosexuality, which would take seriously both the teaching of Scripture and the results of scientific and medical research.'

1.6    Outside the Anglican Communion the position is equally complex. A 'study on sexuality and human relations' entitled *Living in Covenant with God and One Another,* produced for the World Council of Churches by its Family Education Office in 1989, has this to say:

...sexual orientation still represents one of the most painful situations in the arena of sexuality before Christian churches today. The ways in which churches respond vary greatly. Some ignore it, but history and the facts show that it won't go away. Some seek to bury or avoid it, with as little success. Some seek to face it openly, and the result may be turmoil. More and more ... it has become a critical test of faithfulness as churches struggle to know what is God's will for us as sexual beings (Sec. 2.4, page 2 col. 1).

This study also confirms what we said above, that the question of hermeneutics, biblical interpretation, is fundamental to the whole issue:

How do we interpret the words of the Bible as we seek to discover God's Word? ... What set of values do we bring to that interpretation? Is our emphasis on law or on grace? Do we feel that the purity of the faith means that certain people must be excluded, or that its generosity means that all are included and challenged by it? How do we avoid begging the question by the way we ask such questions? (ibid.)

Another significant recent contribution is to be found in Chapter Four of *Human Sexuality,* published in 1990 by the National Conference of Catholic Bishops in the USA. It is important for its pastoral understanding and its concern for new and sensitive language.

1.7    In England 1990 saw the publication of a report to the Methodist Conference by a Commission on Human Sexuality appointed by that Church. We wish to express our appreciation of this document, which is an important contribution for all Christians by reason of its openness to the full range of human experience of sexuality, and the respect with which it reflects on people's personal stories. Its conclusions, however, are in line with those of other contemporary texts, in that it stresses the need for 'a sustained attempt' by the Church 'to come to terms with the issues' before attempting definitive ethical utterance: '... the Church has to live with where the debate is at the moment, and to look to God for the future'. A very similar conclusion was reached by a Working Party of the United Reformed Church, which issued a much briefer Report, specifically on Homosexuality, as a basis for discussion in March 1990.

1.8 We have sought to take account of all these and other current statements, and have been aided by submissions from members of our own House. We have also had the help of gay and lesbian Christians who have generously shared with us their own experiences and concerns. We are grateful to them all. In the event we have felt it right to be more specific and concrete than some other bodies in our guidance to our own Church, but what we say is also offered to all Christians as a contribution to the ecumenical quest for God's will today in this field of human life.

1.9 Our primary aim has been to promote an educational process as a result of which Christians may both become more informed about and understanding of certain human realities, and also enter more deeply into the wisdom of their inheritance of faith in this field. What is needed is unpressured time for prayerful study and reflection, pursued within congregations in whatever ways are most helpful and acceptable and with readiness to listen to those who can speak relevantly from personal experience. Good published material from many points of view is also available. Our hope is that in what follows, while fulfilling our responsibility to address certain practical questions in the immediate situation of our own Church, we can also do something to help forward a general process, marked by greater trust and openness, of Christian reflection on the subject of human sexuality.

# 2. Scripture and Human Sexuality

2.1   When as Christians we consider sexuality or any other aspect of the human condition in the light of Scripture, there are always three distinct realities interacting in our minds and competing for control of our thinking. The first is the content of Scripture itself. The sacred text is diverse, drawn from a period of some twelve centuries, from a wide range of social, cultural and spiritual situations, and influenced by ideas from outside Israel as well as within it. It is possible to discern unifying themes, and to talk in broad terms about a biblical approach to ethics that is centred on God and his covenant-law, the land, the people, their local communities and the family, and about a sexual ethic that is gradually built up within that wider ethical context. But norms of behaviour and the values attaching to the complex roles and relationships of men and women vary from one time and text to another.

2.2   The second reality at work in our thinking will be 'salvation history', that is, the overall shape of the biblical story as this has been perceived by Christian faith and interpreted and told in Christian tradition. In this salvation history the world is created good but then distorted as a result of the decision of free beings to go against the will of God. Chiefly responsible is humankind, made in God's image and likeness, and given power over other creatures as God's steward or viceroy in the world. This human disobedience affects the whole natural order but especially men and women themselves, whose own nature is thereby corrupted and placed in need of liberation from evil. However, the same infinite love which created is also active to rescue and restore. God has been constantly at work to guide history and to support those he loves, and finally in Jesus comes to live in his world in the undistorted image of a humanity perfectly identified with the divine will. In this true humanity he endures all that sin and evil can inflict, and breaks their power by the undefeated love and holiness which pass through the Cross to the Resurrection and Ascension. For those who acknowledge this victorious love of God revealed in Jesus Christ there is forgiveness of sins and access to new and eternal life, in which the transforming presence of God's own Spirit can make every human being Christlike in the way appropriate to each, and ultimately restore the whole creation. This divine work of liberation is seen as foretold or prepared for in various ways by those before Christ who were open to God's mind and message, and as recorded and interpreted for all future generations in the New

Testament. It is as the consistent, reliable and divinely inspired witness to this salvation history that Scripture has been traditionally heard as God's Word, the authoritative revelation of his redeeming purpose and moral will.

2.3   The third component which bears on our approach to Scripture is our general view of the world and our experience of life. In every generation these pose questions which thoughtful Christians seek to answer, and form the background to their understanding as they interpret the Bible for their own day. For many Christians at the present time the world-view they absorb from contemporary western culture, though in many ways open to challenge and increasingly under attack in the course of this century, remains a pervasive influence, particularly inhospitable to biblical ideas. It presents us with a cosmos unimaginably vast and constantly evolving, within which environments such as our own, capable of sustaining life, seem likely to be an infinitesimal minority. We perceive ourselves as both related to and distinct from other developed organisms on this planet, products of genetic mutation and environmental selection. Our understanding of history and of our own personal stories grows ever more complex as we become more aware of the ways in which the lives of communities and individuals are shaped by inheritance and nurture, cultural and economic forces, and biological and geophysical conditions. Within the small and variable margins of human freedom each generation constantly modifies the agreed content of values and norms, of right and wrong. Relationship with God has always been problematic in a world where suffering and deprivation are morally random, but becomes even more so when the intellectual climate is hostile to belief in spiritual reality. In such a chaos of evidence it becomes hard for anyone not already convinced to accept the insights of one faith only as the truth, one set of sacred writings as the fullness of essential revelation, or the moral rules of one small community in the past as normative for everyone for all time.

2.4   Our present discussion is further complicated by the difficulty of defining sexuality in a way that will do justice to all the insights in the wide-ranging contemporary literature on the subject. Rather than become bogged down in a semantic argument that would of necessity be inconclusive, let us instead begin from some of the ordinary-life situations in which human sexual feelings and functions are involved, and note what the Scripture has to say about them.

6

does that imply
it is inexplicable in
un Character

2.5 In the Creation stories humankind is by God's decision both male and female. In Genesis 1 this is the way humanity is made from the first, 'in the image of God...male and female' (v.27). In Genesis 2 the male is created alone, then the female later out of the male body, when other creatures, made by God separately, are found inadequate as partners for the man. In both accounts it is made clear that man and woman are unique among living beings on earth, that they share an equality denied to other creatures, and that they cannot live without each other. In Genesis 2 the man, as a royal figure, has authority over the woman, demonstrated in his giving her her name; but the name also expresses the fact that their natures are essentially the same. The man, from the first, experiences a longing for the woman so powerful that in all generations it will take men away from the parental home to make a new life with their wives; but the woman's relationship to the man is still seen as one which may be called 'subordination-within-equality'. Humankind has a common task and dignity within creation, but the ultimate authority in their partnership is vested in the man. At the same time the importance of both mother and father for the upbringing of children in the family is stressed, and children are taught to pay honour to both (Exod. 20.12; Lev. 19.3; Prov. 1.8-9, 15.20, etc).

2.6 The Bible acknowledges the power of the mutual attraction between men and women, and celebrates it, most notably in the Song of Songs. The strength of a man's love for a woman is classically evoked in a few words in the story of Jacob and Rachel (Gen. 29.20). Proverbs 31 pays tribute to the contribution a woman can make to a domestic, social and economic partnership in the context of a well-to-do family, while the submission considered proper in a wife is reflected in a royal wedding psalm (Ps. 45.11). But Scripture also recognises that sin can disturb the delicate balance of the man-woman partnership. In Genesis 3 part of the woman's punishment for breaking the divinely ordered hierarchy of relations between the sexes by leading the man astray is a desire for him so strong that it makes her his slave, just as the man is punished for abdicating his authority by the rebellion of nature against him. In practice, though Israel was more affirming of women than some other ancient Near Eastern cultures, still there was always what is to the modern mind a severe imbalance in the man-woman relationship. This can be seen, for example, in the husband's technical monopoly of the right to divorce or in the limitations on the part women could take in public worship or community affairs.

7

2.7 The institution of marriage in the Scriptures is closely bound up with the urgent need for sons to preserve the father's name in Israel, to keep secure the family's share in the land, held in trust from God, and to uphold the family honour (cf. Ps. 127.3-5). This, and the fact that to have several wives was a sign of wealth and status, meant that in the early period of Israel's history polygamy was not uncommon, at least amongst the well-off. Even a husband's affection could not make up to a childless wife for the inferiority of her position (1 Sam. 1.1-8).

2.8 Linked with the central importance of procreation is the significance of the male genitals, believed in early times to be the sole source of new life, which was planted complete in the womb by the man's seed. In the stories of the patriarchs an especially solemn oath would be taken with one's hand touching the genitals of the man to whom the promise was made (Gen. 24.2,9). A man whose genitals were damaged or missing was excluded from the worshipping congregation (Deut. 23.1), though in later times a prophet could teach that such a person, if he kept the divine law, would be honoured by God (Isa. 56.4,5).

2.9 On the question of sexual activity outside marriage the Old Testament reflects a slowly evolving morality. As is common in many cultures, a double standard is applied, men having greater freedom than women. That men will have intercourse with their slave-girls is recognised and regulated. Because the woman, whether betrothed or married, is the guarantor of the integrity of the family, adultery is according to the Law punishable by death, though this was often disregarded, and the penalty in time became obsolete. This particular prohibition does, however, play an important role in the teaching of the prophets. The fact that sexual promiscuity was a feature of Canaanite religion, and certainly part of its attraction for those brought up in the austere desert tradition of Israel's faith, led prophets such as Hosea, Jeremiah and Ezekiel to characterise this apostasy as adultery against God, Israel's true husband. To bring out the true horror of the offence, however, they also intensified their language about unfaithfulness, painting the physical act itself as filthy and shameful; and this certainly introduced a new and negative note into biblical references to sexual intercourse. Old Testament society, in short, was no stranger to sexual freedom; and in the second century BC the laments of Ecclesiasticus about the immorality of unmarried daughters, and his warnings against the wiles of loose women on social occasions, confirm that as we

8

approach the New Testament period things have not substantially changed.

2.10    When studied carefully the Old Testament reveals much the same features in its religious attitude to human sexuality as are to be found elsewhere. Sexual desire is recognised as a normal and powerful element in both men and women. It is enjoyed but it is also suspect as in some way incompatible with holiness in particular. A soldier fighting for the God of Israel is expected to abstain from intercourse. The genitals are both sacred and shameful. Sexual feeling is by no means seen only in terms of procreation, but the social significance of the latter, intensified by the central importance for Israelites of ancestral rights in the Promised Land, leads to strenuous legal and educational efforts to regulate sexual relations. Out of all this emerges in time a generous human ideal, that of the monogamous, faithful couple, where husband and wife remain together into old age and even though they are childless (cf., e.g., Mal. 2 13-16; Luke 1.5-7). Marriage becomes for some a spiritual as well as a physical and social partnership, a state to be entered into with prayer for the divine blessing and for the grace of mutual faithfulness (Tobit 8.4-9).

2.11    It is against the background of this human and ethical development that references to other manifestations of sexuality are to be evaluated. A passage such as Leviticus 18, for example, lists a variety of activities which are characterised as 'shame', 'lewdness', 'uncleanness', 'abomination', and so forth. These include such diverse matters as intercourse within the family, whether with relatives by blood or by marriage, intercourse with a woman during her menstrual period, adultery (with the wife of another Israelite), male homosexual intercourse, and bestiality. All these things are condemned first because they violate holiness and ritual purity, and secondly because they are behaviour typical of the Canaanites whom God dispossessed to give the land to his people. If Israel also practises these things which God finds abominable, they too will be punished in the same way. Such catalogues make quite clear that Israel and its neighbours were familiar as we are with widely varying forms of sexual desire and conduct. In Leviticus 20 death is the prescribed penalty for each case in a similar list of offences.

2.12    In discussions of the scriptural view of human sexuality reference is also commonly made to an early story concerning Sodom. In Genesis 19.5 the men of Sodom surround Lot's house and call upon Lot to bring

9

out his angelic visitors 'that we may know them', usually interpreted in a sexual sense. Some commentators have suggested that the sin which the men of Sodom committed was to breach the hospitality that Lot was extending to his guests, and that 'know' here means simply to examine someone's credentials. However, the use of the same verb with what is unmistakably the sexual meaning three verses later must be decisive for the interpretation. All that can properly be said is that there is a threatened violation of hospitality consisting in homosexual rape, and that this is condemned as 'wicked'. This reading is supported by the similar story set in Gibeah, where the same phraseology is used (Judges 19.16ff): 'Bring out the man who came into your house that we may know him', to which the owner of the house replies, 'Do not act so wickedly...do not do this vile thing'. In both instances the offer or sacrifice of a woman as an alternative sexual victim confirms the understanding that rape is intended. Ezekiel 16. 49-50 characterises the 'iniquity of Sodom' as a selfish pride which, despite great affluence, refused to help the poor in their need (cf. perhaps Isa. 1.10-17). Other references, both in the Old and in the New Testament, are couched in general terms (Isa. 3.9; Matt. 11. 23f). Sodom certainly became a stock image for extreme sinfulness, incurring sudden and annihilating judgement (Isa. 1.9; 13.19; Lam. 4.6; Amos 4.11; Matt. 10.15; Luke 17.29 etc.), but not, it would seem, a symbol for one particular sin – though Jude 7 makes specific a more general reference in 2 Peter 2.6-7.

2.13.  In the New Testament the Judaistic background is the product of the general development noted in the Old. The ethical ideal is that sexual activity is to be confined within faithful, heterosexual marriage, normally lifelong, and Jesus is recorded as upholding this in his own teaching (Mark 10.1-12; Matt. 5.31-32; 19.3-9; cf. Luke 16.18; 1 Cor. 10-11). The man is the dominant partner; family – the perpetuation of the father's name in Israel (note the surprise in Luke 1.61) – is the key concern. Attitudes to adultery and prostitution have already been mentioned. Alongside all this, however, other notes are also sounded. The idea, found earlier, for example, in the story of Jeremiah, that sexual activity is incompatible with total dedication to the cause of God is definitely present. John the Baptist is one instance. Jesus's invitation to those who feel capable of the sacrifice to make themselves eunuchs for the sake of the Kingdom of Heaven is another. Paul continues the theme in the light of his expectation that the Last Day will soon come (1 Cor. 7.29-35). But neither Jesus nor Paul demands celibacy as a condition of

Christian discipleship, as certain sects were later to do. Paul indeed explicitly recognises the strength of sexual desire, and regards marriage as the one divinely ordained place for its physical expression (1 Cor.7. 1-9), though he sees celibacy as a better state in which to serve the Lord (1 Cor.7. 35-38). In all this there are clear rules for conduct, but no actual denigration of marriage. What there is also, however, is a conscious focusing, in Paul especially but not exclusively, on breach of the sexual rules as one of the sins most likely to endanger the security of salvation for Christians.

2.14    The reason for this specific anxiety is almost certainly to be found in the greater sexual licence of the Gentile world compared with that of Judaism (cf., e.g., 1 Peter 4.3-5). The sexual behaviour of Hellenistic culture included, of course, a well-known element of homosexual activity by both sexes but principally by men. The New Testament makes reference to this in four documents: in three letters of Paul, and in Jude. Of these passages that in the first chapter of Romans is by far the most important.

2.15    Paul follows a line of argument known to us from other Jewish writers, namely that the worship of idols is the origin and cause of every evil. Human beings ought to have been able to arrive at knowledge of God the Creator and of his character from contemplation of his works; but because they upset right order by giving mere creatures the worship due only to God, they themselves were abandoned to disorder in their own selves, so that they misdirected and misused their most intimate and personal feelings. 'For this reason God gave them up to dishonourable passions. Their women exchanged natural relations for unnatural; their men likewise gave up natural relations with women and were consumed with passion for one another, men committing shameless acts with men' (vv. 26 and 27). There is particular significance in the two words 'dishonourable passions'. Paul takes for granted an ordering of things in which the body and its sexual desires have their place and their proper honour; but the sexual acts of which he is now speaking dishonour the body. Passions are more than emotions; they are emotions out of control. Dishonourable passions are a disordering of God's purpose. In 1 Corinthians 6, among the categories of the unrighteous who, Paul says, will not inherit the Kingdom of God are the *malakoi* and the *arsenokoitai*, words usually held to denote men who adapt passive and active roles in homosexual intercourse respectively. In 1 Timothy 1.9,10 the word

11

*arsenokoitai* is also used in a list of those whose activities break the law and offend the Gospel.

2.16 Did the ancient world recognise a class of people who were homosexual by orientation? The phenomenon of homosexual activity in ancient Greek civilisation was complex. In classical times, for example, adult males, alongside their lives as husbands and fathers, engaged in relations with youths in early puberty (not children) which were not simply sexual in content but carried social and cultural significance, and were governed by strict conventions. At the same time society recognised the existence of those, predominantly male, who appeared to be attracted entirely to members of their own sex; and both this and homosexual prostitution continued down into the early New Testament period. Such relationships were often condemned. It was held, for example, to the credit of the philosopher Plato that, though attracted to members of his own sex, he did not engage in physical relationships. It can be said, therefore, that phenomena which today would be interpreted in terms of orientation were present and recognised. But the modern concept of orientation has been developed against a background of genetic and psychological theory which was not available to the ancient world.

2.17 At the same time the Bible has a positive approach to the possibilities of affection in same-sex relationships. Expressions of the depth of affection between one man and another, or one woman and another, can have the quality of similar affection within the marriage bond. Ruth and Naomi ('Where you go I will go; and where you lodge I will lodge': Ruth 1.16) and David and Jonathan ('Your love to me was wonderful, passing the love of women': 2 Sam. 1.26) are good examples, to say nothing of the warmth of affection between Jesus and his disciples, or the injunctions to brotherly love in the New Testament letters. The theory has sometimes been advanced that Jesus himself was homosexual, either in orientation or even in practice. To this it must be replied that the New Testament offers no evidence to justify such a conclusion; and that neither his opponents in his own day nor hostile writers in the period of the early Church who attack him on other charges make any mention of any kind of sexual behaviour. It has also been remarked that we have no record of any explicit teaching by Jesus on the subject of homosexual relations. This is true. But from the fact that he supports with his own authority the statement in Genesis that in the beginning God created

12

humankind male and female, and uses that as a basis for ethical guidance (Matt. 19. 3-9; Mark 10.1-12), it is not unreasonable to infer that he regarded heterosexual love as the God-given pattern.

2.18   How are we to evaluate this scriptural material? To begin with we can recognise human experience that we share: the power of sexual love; the joy of being in love; the blessing of a good lifelong union; the temptation to unfaithfulness or to multiple relationships; the phenomenon of prostitution. The issue of subordination or equality in a man-woman sexual partnership is a question for us today, as are the roles of mother and father in the upbringing of children. Conventions about modesty still exercise us. The pain of childlessness is as real as it was then. So are the spiritual dimension of the marriage covenant and the renunciation of marriage for a life of service. To all these situations the people of the Bible speak in ways that enable us to relate our experience to theirs and, if we will, to learn from it.

2.19   In the same way we can approach what the Bible has to say on these matters with the faith-pattern of salvation history, and learn from that dialogue. Thus the story of the Fall may not be a literally historical account of human development but it still points us to fundamental truths of our condition. We can and should acknowledge the goodness of God's primal gifts, emerging from the evolutionary creation for which he is responsible, and including in the present context the fact of gender and the potential for fullness of sexual life and relationships, for procreation, family and human society and civilisation. In the same way we have to face the reality of the counterforce of sin and evil, which may be rooted in our fragile nature but which has also been intensified by human culture in all periods.

2.20   Furthermore we can acknowledge and be grateful for the corrective responses to evil and the creative visions of goodness and hope which God has inspired most especially in the spiritual life of Israel. We can and should receive these not as each individually the totality of relevant truth but as cumulatively a God-given guide and as the necessary preparation for God's key act of revelation and liberation in Christ. In the New Testament we have the unique treasure both of the fourfold Gospel presentation of that divine redemptive act and of the Spirit-guided reflections upon it for faith and discipleship of those who were closest to the first coming of the Lord.

2.21   One cardinal point that salvation history should make clear to us is that Scripture provides its own criterion for judging its various contents. This criterion is what St Paul calls 'the mind of Christ'. For Christians today this will include partly the teaching and example of Jesus as recorded in the Gospels, and partly the guidance in the rest of the New Testament which came from reflection on the person and work of Christ by the leaders of the earliest Church. But that is not all. This latter reflection was itself carried on in the light given by God's own Spirit; and this process continues in each generation as the Church seeks to discover the mind of Christ for its own moral and spiritual needs. The Spirit guides the Church in learning from the dialogue between Scripture and contemporary circumstance. To this dialogue any part of Scripture may contribute; but where there is a genuine difference in ethical understanding between the New Testament and the Old, it is from the New Testament that the Church must derive its controlling interpretation.

2.22   At any given time we also feed into this Spirit-led dialogue our own world view and our awareness of new circumstances. The result may be one of two things or a mixture of both. In some cases the message of Scripture will judge our contemporary views, showing up their superficiality or wrong-headedness. But where new factors or new understandings make our situation significantly different from that of the biblical writers, Scripture may guide us more by stimulating new perceptions in us than by giving direction that can be applied as it stands. Christian ethical thinking on modern economic problems is one obvious example of a field in which this latter approach is relevant.

2.23   The stories of Sodom and Gibeah mentioned earlier illustrate both these points. It would be legitimate to find in these episodes authority for condemning gang rape, or mob violence against visiting foreigners. These are situations very close to the original incident, and the lesson is wholly in accord with the New Testament. It would clearly not be legitimate to say that they justify a host in offering his daughter to the mob to save his guests, or an intended victim in sacrificing a woman with whom he was cohabiting to save himself. Anyone can see for themselves that such actions are not compatible with the mind of Christ. What, however, Christians have too often failed to see is that these stories simply are not relevant to the case, say, of two men or two women who find themselves deeply emotionally attracted to one another, and who

14

wish to live together in a sexual relationship for mutual support in every area of their lives. The situations are too far apart in human terms for any ethical transfer to be made.

2.24 The situation with regard to the Old Testament Law is rather more subtle. Mainstream Christianity has always recognised the authority of many of the ethical commands of the Old Testament. Thus the Thirty-nine Articles of Religion lay down that while Christians are not bound by the ceremonial, ritual and civil laws of the Old Testament no one is free from the commandments which are called 'moral' (Article 7). Some have recently argued that prohibitions such as those in Leviticus 18 or 20 do not come under the category of moral law but relate simply to requirements for cultic purity, and therefore no longer apply in the Christian dispensation. This argument is unsound in several respects. To begin with, requirements for admission to the cult in Israel were not confined to matters of ritual purity. Much of the thrust of the prophets' teaching was directed precisely to the point that the worshipper needed to have hands that were morally as well as ceremonially clean; and the same principle is reflected in the Law, the Psalms and the Wisdom writings. The fact that a regulation is found, for example, in the laws of holiness which have a strong cultic context does not determine whether or not it counts as 'moral' for us. God himself, the Holy One of Israel, Isaiah says, 'reveals his holiness by righteousness' (5.16). That part of Leviticus which has as its theme the necessity for Israel to be holy because the Lord who is in the midst of them is holy mixes up together a wide variety of commands: dietary regulations or laws against occult practices appear alongside rules for honesty in commerce or injunctions to honour the old and to love as yourself even the foreigner who lives in your community. The fact is that the Old Testament does not make distinctions between moral goodness and ritual purity in the way Christians came to do after the destruction of the Temple and the end of the ancient cult. Holiness for the Old Testament is all-embracing, and we have to make our own decisions in the light of Christ as to what parts of the old Law still have guidance for us and in what way.

2.25 When we do this, we exercise a large liberty in the Spirit. Many Old Testament laws relating to the offering of sacrifices, for example, are simply no longer relevant, for Christ has put an end to the sacrificial cult by the one offering of himself, once for all. At the same time we still need to approach God in worship with the reverence and awe and purity

15

of heart which those laws were meant to ensure. Thanks to the Gospel we no longer need a priest to be our intermediary with God, for we are in Christ, and his Spirit in us enables each one of us to call on God direct as 'Abba', 'Father'. But the other face of that coin is that we are all members of a royal priesthood, and as such are challenged by the Old Testament Law to live in the holiness that becomes that vocation. Our bodies are to be 'temples of the Holy Spirit' (1 Cor.6.19). It is for us to decide in the light of the Gospel what that holiness involves. We shall not follow the Old Testament in saying, for instance, that someone who has been helping at the scene of an accident, and there has touched a dead body, cannot therefore come that same day to receive Holy Communion. But we shall say, as the Book of Common Prayer lays down, that communicants must be truly and earnestly penitent for sin, in love and charity with their neighbours, and committed to the new life in Christ which keeps God's commands and walks in his ways.

2.26   The crux of the matter, therefore, so far as sexuality is concerned, is whether the sexual behaviour in the life-style of an individual or group is holy in itself and conducive to growth in holiness. For Christians the primary definition of holiness will be whatever is in accord with the spirit of Christ and promotes Christlikeness. When we ask what is Christlike in the field of sexuality, however, we cannot answer simply in terms of the actual sexual practice of the historical Jesus, for the simple reason that the Jesus shown to us in the Gospels is unmarried and Christian holiness has always included the married state, as it did with the Apostle Peter. Fundamentally holiness in the New Testament is concerned with the fruits of the Spirit and obedience to the will of God. These things show themselves in qualities and dispositions, such as those listed by St Paul in Galatians 5.22 ff., Philippians 4.8 or 1 Corinthians 13, and in the performance of good actions and the avoidance of sinful ones. Those whose lives are of this kind are those who truly love both God and neighbour.

2.27   It may be helpful also to say something at this point about the relation between the concepts of sin and divine law. In one application of the term 'sin' any dispositions, feelings, thoughts or actions that are contrary to the will and purpose of God are sinful, and those who yield to them or carry them out are sinners or commit sin. In another usage, however, the language of 'sin' refers to wrong consciously and deliberately done and, strictly speaking, wrong recognised as violating

16

the divine will. Thus, before Paul can say that 'all have sinned and are deprived of the glory of God' (Rom.3.23), he is at pains to show both that there has been law to make people aware that they are doing wrong, and that such law is universal, revealed in Scripture to the Jews but also accessible to the Gentiles through reasoned reflection on experience. Both usages are acknowledged later in the same Letter to the Romans, when he writes: 'Sin was already in the world before there was law; and although in the absence of law no reckoning is kept of sin, death held sway from Adam to Moses, even over those who had not sinned as Adam did, by disobeying a direct command' (Rom.5.13-14, REB). It is important in discussion, therefore, to be careful not to slide without explanation from one use of 'sin' terminology to the other. 'Sin' in the narrower sense implies both understanding in the agent of its sinfulness and deliberate choice on the agent's part. An action may be contrary to God's will; it may witness to that 'original sin' whereby, as Article 9 says we are 'very far gone from original righteousness'; but it will not make the doer guilty of actual sin unless there is at least some awareness of its wrong character and some free consent of the individual's own will to what is done. The point is of importance for our present discussion. In considering sexual lifestyles some Christians have always felt it important to characterise particular behaviour as sinful in itself, because it is contrary to the divine norms. Others have preferred to concentrate on the situation and convictions of the agents, and to ask whether they are guilty of witting and deliberate sin. Because of this ambiguity we have in the present document made little use of the specific term 'sin', lest it should lead to misunderstanding in certain contexts. But we believe it will be clear where we regard this or that type of conduct as objectively contrary to the will of God, and in what circumstances we consider free moral agents to be guilty of sinful behaviour.

2.28    When we reflect on Paul's teaching in Romans 1 in the light of all these considerations, it is clear first that he follows the Old Testament Law in regarding all homosexual practice as sinful in itself, and also that he is interpreting this conduct in terms of the good and evil impulses which play such a significant part in rabbinic understanding of the human moral predicament. Such behaviour is for him an expression of the evil impulse in human beings. God, he says, has removed from those Gentiles who have this particular desire the good impulse that would have helped them to resist it, and so has abandoned them to sin in retribution for their folly in worshipping idols. Hence this is not the only evil now let loose

17

among them; indeed there is no wickedness to which they are not addicted. Their ultimate depravity is that they know that all this wrongdoing will bring on them just destruction from God, and yet they do not care, but call evil good. There are a number of points to be made about this passage, particularly about the concept of 'nature', which we shall have to address later. For the moment we need to note the question raised by Paul's aetiology of homosexual practice. How does this relate, say, to the young man or woman, baptised, confirmed, communicant, converted and committed to personal faith in Christ and to holiness in life, perhaps longing to be ordained or commissioned to particular Christian ministry, who find themselves to be attracted strongly and only to those of the same sex, and in their own conscientious judgement unable to attain inner peace or stability until that fact is accepted positively? We have deliberately taken a real-life case at the opposite pole from Paul's picture. To do so is not to deny that there may be cases to which Paul's words are appropriate. But the differences between such cases and the one we have cited are one measure of the problem we face in seeking light from Scripture in this complex area of human sexuality.

2.29   There is, therefore, in Scripture an evolving convergence on the ideal of lifelong, monogamous, heterosexual union as the setting intended by God for the proper development of men and women as sexual beings. Sexual activity of any kind outside marriage comes to be seen as sinful, and homosexual practice as especially dishonourable. It is also recognised that God may call some to celibacy for particular service in his cause. Only by living within these boundaries are Christians to achieve that holiness which is pleasing to God. As we have already noted, this ultimate biblical consensus presents us with certain problems which need to be faced. But it is quite clearly the foundation on which the Church's traditional teaching is built, and it is to that teaching we must next turn.

# 3. The Christian Vision for Human Sexuality

3.1   It would seem appropriate at this point to set out an account of the Christian ideal or vision for human sexuality as this has developed within the context just described. Because sexual love is a wonderful gift from God, then through it, if all goes well, a man and a woman can be united in a relationship which for depth, intensity and joy is unique in their experience. They can find a strength and support in one another which helps each of them to mature as individuals. They can form a partnership which is both a blessing to the whole community and also the stable and loving environment in which children need to be brought up. Being much more than simply physical organisms, they share their lives with one another at many different levels – bodily, emotional, intellectual, social and spiritual. To share at the bodily level alone is to make a relationship far less than it could be. But the body makes a unique contribution. Because full sexual relations are intimate, and can be ecstatically happy, they can make the partners supremely precious to one another, and so help them to treasure their sharing at all other levels. In this way an incomparable union can be built on the physical foundation.

3.2   Because of this affirmation of the body one basic principle is very definitely implicit in Christian thinking about sexual relations. It may be put this way: the greater the degree of personal intimacy, the greater should be the degree of personal commitment. This is in fact true to much human experience. Often it is only because a relationship has advanced to a point of deep trust, valuing and commitment that inhibitions and privateness are surrendered, and intercourse becomes a welcomed possibility. For Christian tradition this has been, as it were, codified in the principle that full sexual intercourse requires total commitment, that is, in the words of the marriage service, 'faithful' and 'forsaking all others' 'to have and to hold ... for better, for worse, for richer, for poorer, in sickness and in health, to love and to cherish, till death us do part'. It has to be recognised, however, that our society today has very largely abandoned this Christian definition of the degree of commitment there ought to be, and we find a wide range of situations. For a growing number their first experience of full intercourse will come soon after puberty, both in a desire to experiment and also in a process of self-discovery through sharing oneself with another. Later on sexual relations

19

may be seen as a source of pleasure and satisfaction which it is right for people to enjoy, and those who want to enjoy it together are considered entitled to do so. For others there has to be personal friendship and loyalty, including fidelity for the time of the relationship, but with no requirement of permanence, which may or may not come later. There is also a whole range of relationships which have some reference, direct or indirect, positive or negative, to the institution of marriage. A couple may be lovers, and share much of their lives, but not live together, though the option of doing so eventually is tacitly or explicitly present. Others will live exactly as if married, but refuse to enter into the formal and public marriage relationship. Another couple may agree on a trial marriage, regarding actual marriage and possible parenthood as something that should not be undertaken without some assurance that the parties are compatible. Another couple may be quite clear that they intend to marry, but housing problems or other constraints seem to make that impracticable for the present. On a rather different spectrum there are lovers who may sustain a faithful relationship for years, but for reasons ranging from careers to bad personal experiences in the past cannot bring themselves to marry, or lovers who find themselves thrown together in situations of loneliness, stress or danger, and in even a short relationship find the human support they need. In all these instances, and many more that could be quoted, a proportion between physical intimacy and personal commitment is always present but varying widely from case to case. To this complex human situation, which in whole or in part constantly recurs in history, Christian teaching about marriage offers something much better than what it is commonly taken to be, namely a regulation which simply condemns those who break it. It offers two things: first, guidance, based on God's revelation in Scripture and Christian experience, as to the way of life within which full physical expression of our sexuality can best contribute to our own maturity and sanctification and that of others; and secondly, a direction in which other sexual relationships can and should move, if they are to serve more effectually the true fulfilment of those concerned.

3.3   Speaking specifically now of marriage, this fulfilment, both of the individual partners and of their partnership, will not come without cost, hard work and self-denial. A true marriage reflects Christ's own love for us all. He too gave himself to others 'for better, for worse, till death'. In it we learn to break down our pride and self-concern, to be open to our partner as he or she really is, to treasure what is good and forgive faults, to sacrifice ourselves for the sake of the other, to be loyal whatever the price. In these ways marriage becomes a means of grace, making us more like Christ both in ourselves and in our dealings with the world around us.

3.4 Nowadays many claim that this total and unconditional mutual commitment which is the heart of the Christian understanding of marriage is a restrictive bondage into which no one can be expected to enter. Marriage, they say, should be seen as a contract, to be ended if it falls short of what we expect. But such freedom is of much less worth than the freedom which faithfulness brings – the security within which to face our faults and grow out of them for love's sake. What may seem bondage from a self-centred point of view is a miracle of liberation when seen from the other end: that this person we love so much is prepared to take us on, with all our faults, for life. A good marriage creates for each partner the same kind of environment which we recognise as promoting growth to maturity in the case of children: a combination of love and challenge within an unbreakably reliable relationship.

3.5 We need to guard, however, against the idea that marriage is a purely private, inward-looking arrangement – 'selfishness for two' or, where there are children, for three or four or whatever the number may be. The prayers in the ASB Marriage Service ask for the couple 'grace to minister to others' and to be 'by deed and word ... witnesses of your saving love to those among whom they live'. By this witness 'in this troubled world' they are to enable unity to overcome division, forgiveness to heal injury, and joy to triumph over sorrow. A married couple are not simply to serve each other but to stand side by side in service to the world; and it is the strength of their many-dimensioned partnership which will make them more effective means of grace together than they could have been apart. Just as a wedding is a public ceremony, so a marriage is a public fact. It is a re-shaping of human life within the community, and as such has a responsibility to the community to be a force for good in its life.

3.6 It is also the marriage committed to loving stability which alone can provide the best home for our children. There is no such thing as a marriage breakdown in which the children do not suffer, even if the marriage has been far from perfect. Teachers and social workers alike report that where a child has behavioural problems a home broken or at risk of breakdown is the factor that features in the story more often than any other. The child's tragedy begins with the lack of total commitment to the marriage on the part of one or both parents.

3.7    It is as supporting and encouraging men and women to make their own all the good that lifelong marriage can provide that we are best to understand the strength of the teaching against divorce and remarriage which in the New Testament Mark, Luke and Paul attribute to Jesus. The word of Christ is the true wisdom: 'That which God has joined' – i.e. the marriage relationship – 'let not man put asunder' (Mark 10.9). In Matthew Jesus is said to have made an exception for cases where the wife had been guilty of adultery (Matt. 5.32; 19.9), but the exact context and significance of this exceptive ruling is still matter for scholarly debate. Paul in 1 Cor. 7.12-16 admits a further exception in the case of marriage between a Christian and a non-Christian, where the non-Christian asks for a divorce. But such marginal relaxations do not significantly alter the force of teaching which Jesus bases on the purpose of God in creation, as presented in the account in Genesis 2 referred to earlier.

3.8    For all these positive reasons God's perfect will for married people is chastity before marriage, and then a lifelong relationship of fidelity and mutual sharing at all levels. We recognise that it is increasingly hard today for the unmarried generally, and for young people facing peer group pressure in particular, to hold to this ideal, and therefore both the Church and its individual members need to be clearer and stronger in supporting those who are struggling against the tide of changing sexual standards. But, if we believe in a Gospel of grace and restoration freely offered to all, we need to give this support in such a way that those who may eventually go with that tide will not feel that in the Church's eyes they are from then on simply failures for whom there is neither place nor love in the Christian community. It is by focussing our teaching on the positive value of the Christian vision for human life that we shall best avoid this danger.

3.9    For the majority of human beings marriage, in many cultures at quite an early age, is the normal pattern. But there are also all those who never marry, or who do so late in life. What is God's will for the single person?

3.10    The first thing the Christian will want to say to the single is that

*This is surely a dangerous way to proceed — it is clearly a-textual as ideal?*

Jesus himself was single. Any idea that to be unmarried is to fall short as a human being is totally false. On the contrary, the heart of what it is to be human was shown to us in one who never married. No true disciple of Christ can accept the fashionable opinion of our times that experience of full physical sex relations is necessary for our fulfilment as human beings. Our Lord himself and many of his greatest saints have been living proof that this is not so. At the same time our sexuality, male or female, has a great and permanent part to play in the life of each one of us. We are men or women in everything we do, and we should enjoy the colour and delight, the strength and sensitivity this brings, and which is one of God's loveliest gifts.

3.11   There are many reasons why people may live in the single state. Some choose it for its privacy or independence; some accept it as a condition of their work or of responsibility to care for dependants; for others it may be the result of disability or difficulty with relationships; for others again it is simply their sad experience that, for whatever reason, the person they could and would have loved and married, and who could and would have loved and married them, has never entered their lives. At least 50 per cent of married people at some stage find themselves single again through bereavement, when they have to cope on their own with the burden of grief as well. It is all too easy to make single people feel excluded or diminished when, for example, Christians talk, preach or write as though everyone must be married or live in a family. We need to ask ourselves whether the Church always gives the same prayerful attention to the human and spiritual needs of single people as it commonly does to the married or those in the religious life. Can we honestly say that every congregation is a fellowship in which hidden loneliness is discerned, or where those without natural groups to support them are readily welcomed into sensitive and appropriate circles of companionship?

3.12   Many of the most valuable contributions to work or community are made by single people who can go to places or undertake tasks which those with family responsibilities cannot contemplate, or who have time and energy to devote in all kinds of ways to the needs of others. One special gift which the single, if they will, have the freedom to develop is that of friendship. Jesus says to his closest followers, 'I have called you friends' (John 15.15), and the Gospels show him as one who had this gift of being friends with a wide variety of people. Friendship is undervalued in

23

the present age, indeed its potentialities are far from fully understood. The word 'friend', like 'neighbour', used to have a much wider reference than it does today. It included colleagues, fellow workers, and members of one's social or occupational group. Most warm and collaborative relationships with people of either sex, for instance in sport or leisure, are varieties of friendship. In particular cultures and periods of history friendships have also had a much richer emotional quality than our own time feels comfortable to allow them. Reference has already been made to the biblical story of David and Jonathan. Later Christian tradition too contains many wonderful examples of these deep friendships. We see them in the lives of men like Basil the Great, Augustine or Aelred of Rievaulx, or in the partnership of Francis de Sales and Jane Frances de Chantal. Our own day is much too ready to interpret any intimate friendship as no more than a disguise for hidden homosexual or heterosexual involvement, a tendency which can not only inflict hurt but also actively inhibit the development of friendship in general.

3.13    True friendship, like marriage, calls for loyalty. It involves sharing at many levels. It too is a means of grace for the growth of our personalities. It can greatly enhance the quality of our work or of our general service of others. At the same time it is more flexible than marriage. It can more easily tolerate parting, and pick up again after a lapse of time. Above all, friendship, however deep, is never exclusive.

3.14    This is the fundamental reason why full physical sexual relations, or behaviour that would normally and naturally lead to such relations, have no place in friendship or, indeed, in the life of the single person in general. The proper fulfilment of such relations, the good which they serve, is that of unique lifelong commitment to one partner. Where such commitment is not possible, the effect of the physical relationship is not in the end to enhance life for those concerned but to impair it. It frustrates both parties because their love can never achieve the purpose at all levels for which God intends it. It is especially important that young people should be helped to understand this and to realise the importance of the art of friendship with both sexes. The young need the fun and support of the sympathetic peer group without the premature pairing off into intense relationships which our culture endlessly urges upon them. In fact everyone of every age needs to learn how to be and to have friends. Friendship between husband and wife is a vital element within the married state itself; and it is also important that marriage partners should

24

have friends other than their spouse, and not be totally dependent for human enrichment on each other. But all this can flourish only within the framework of chastity.

3.15    It is important to distinguish the single state in general from that of celibacy, with which in common parlance it is today often confused. The single state may be the individual's preference or it may not; it may be the time before marriage, or after being widowed or, increasingly in our own contemporary culture, after being divorced. The single state becomes celibacy only when it is freely and deliberately chosen 'in order to devote oneself completely to God and his concerns'. Our Lord's single life, therefore, was one of celibacy; and many Christians down the centuries have been inspired to follow him in that life in their quest for Christlikeness. It is, however, increasingly recognised in the Churches today that celibacy is a special gift and calling of the Holy Spirit, in accordance with Jesus's own words in Matthew 19.12: 'For while some are incapable of marriage because they were born so, or were made so by men, there are others who have renounced marriage for the sake of the Kingdom of Heaven. Let those accept who can' (REB). Celibacy is thus a choice of the unmarried state not for self-regarding reasons but from love in order to be able to serve God and neighbour more freely, whether through the life of prayer or through activity or both. To prescribe 'celibacy', therefore, for all those for whom marriage, for whatever reason, is impossible is a misuse of the term. Celibacy cannot be prescribed for anyone. What is needed is that the single should live in the form of chastity appropriate to their situation.

3.16    All three ways of life which we have described – the married, the single and the celibate – are ones which by the grace of God can help to transform our fallen human nature. Marriage being a part of God's good gift in creation, both the married state and others which are defined in relation to it can have this power for good in all human life, wherever they are inspired by the same values and ideals, and can be a means of advancing the Kingdom of God. At the same time failure to acknowledge these values and ideals and to be guided by them or toward them is a plentiful source of disorder and suffering. The bogus philosophies of erotic freedom which have, for example, marked twentieth century European culture, and which have sought to justify every excess or deviation, stand condemned by the chaos and misery, disease and death they have brought into many lives.

25

3.17 If sexuality is a great blessing, it is also a dangerous one. To begin with, in order to ensure the survival of the species, sexual feelings need generally to be very strong. If the mortality of each is not to result in the death of all, then there has to be some drive that will transcend the limited interests of each individual for the sake of a future beyond its grasp. But this impulse is part of a sexuality which is in various ways defective or distorted or corrupted, because it is linked at a profound level with our whole personality and identity. In theological terms we are fallen creatures. The 'image of God' in us is not wholly defaced, but there is nothing in us which is not in some degree marred, disordered, out of true. When, therefore, the strong forces of sexuality are caught up in this disorder, which may be physical as well as spiritual, the effects are complex and far-reaching, and can be very destructive.

3.18 These effects take a wide variety of forms. For some, sex brings full satisfaction only when the other person is unwilling or frightened, or when it takes the form of rape or abuse, perhaps of the old or very young. Others find pleasure chiefly in seduction or adultery, or in using sex as a means of emotional blackmail or manipulation. For a tiny minority the compulsion may be to intercourse with animals or even the dead. Sex may become simply one way of demonstrating power, subjugation or revenge, as in the violation of prisoners or of occupied civilian populations in war. To the pimp or brothel-keeper it is a means of making money while enjoying the satisfaction of humiliating and degrading others. Again, sexual feelings may be stimulated by a wide range of situations. For some, physical relations are difficult or even impossible without either inflicting or enduring pain. In others the stimulus may be a material object or the sight of other people engaging in a particular sexual practice. Some can find release only in fantasies acted out on their own or while watching films and videos or listening to 'hot' telephone lines or reading pornographic literature. Historically and today sexual activity has been linked with occultism and various forms of black magic.

3.19 Human sexuality is a very fragile system, easily distorted or broken. There have always been a certain number of both men and women who find genital sex very difficult or even impossible, and others whose sexuality feels to them at odds with their bodies, so that they become convinced of their need for sex change, or enter the world of the transvestite. Damage to sexuality, sometimes irreversible, can be done very early in life. The personality is given a twist which puts normal sex out of reach. Furthermore, because sexual pleasure is intense, equalled perhaps only by that of certain drugs, costs nothing and is constantly available, it can easily become a prop which the personality cannot do without.

3.20 The intensity and availability of sexual pleasure, combined with the fact of the complex needs within the psyche which find relief or satisfaction through its many expressions, have given it also especial significance for human spirituality. In all ages some have seen in sexual ecstasy an entry into the realm of the divine, or have made sexual activity a ritual for securing divine blessing on human life. The Judaeo-Christian tradition has from Old Testament times onwards been implacably opposed to this divinisation of sex. Although erotic imagery has been one appropriate way of describing mystical union through prayer, there has also in Christian spirituality been a cautiousness about erotic pleasure. Because 'being in love' is all pervasive, driving other concerns to the margins of attention, and because love-making is an authentically ecstatic experience, excluding everything else from consciousness, the Church has tended to see sexual attraction and activity as particularly hostile to God's due place as the supreme object of human love and the proper controller of all human thought, feeling and conduct.

3.21 Awareness of these factors has repeatedly led the Church to adopt a repressive attitude to sexual desire in its teaching, and to present it as something to be tolerated as a necessity but feared as an easy occasion for mortal sin and as having no place in perfect holiness. Within that tradition the virtue of chastity has at times been defined either as absolute abstinence with a refusal to allow erotic thoughts and feelings to lodge in the conscious mind, or as strict control of the emotions even within a totally faithful marriage relationship. There is no doubt that fear and guilt have also played a large part both in the way this teaching has been put across and in its effects on those who have received it. But equally there have been many in every generation who have found joy and fulfilment, whether in the married or single state, in a life which has affirmed the emotions and yet has been faithful to Christian ideals. In modern western Christianity, largely in response to secular developments in the study of human psychology, this more positive ideal of chastity has been strengthened to emphasise thankfulness to God for human feelings and to acknowledge how much they have to contribute to the quality of personal relationships. Instead of an anxious tabu on physical contacts, for example, the ideal is for a style which is more natural and spontaneous but which respects the integrity of the individual by not crossing the boundaries beyond which full erotic relationships lie. Nevertheless, experience shows that this balance is not easy to achieve, and firm standards of self-discipline and self-denial are as necessary as they have always been if sexuality is to be channelled within the bounds of God's kind of love for our neighbour.

3.22    But though secular developments have in some respects had a healthy influence, in others they have been destructive of much possible human happiness, and Christians have not been immune from these effects. In particular, western society today has become widely obsessed with sexual pleasure as an end in itself and almost, it seems at times, as an inalienable human right. This over-emphasis on one particular good thing can cause needless and even tragic human misery by destroying the sense of self-worth in those who either lack strong sexual desires or have sexual difficulties, by encouraging premature sex experience outside marriage and infidelity within it, and by undermining relationships which could be stable and satisfying if the other blessings they bring were given proper weight.

3.23    What the 1928 Prayer Book called the need for 'the natural instincts and affections' to be 'hallowed and directed aright' is something that cannot be met without the taking up of the Cross. Simply trying to rehabilitate marriage as an institution will not achieve what is needed, for marriage is no more than ordinary human beings trying to live in the state they believe marriage to be, and both they and their perceptions need redemption. It is vital to recognise that most marriages are bound to fall short in varying degrees of the ideal we have described earlier, and not to succumb to another fantasy of our culture, the sentimental dream of an idyllic, romantic union in which the failings, sins and incompatibilities that mark us all are magically done away. Marriage even in a good world would call for sacrifice. Even more in the world as it is, it cannot be simply an experience of fulfilment, but must involve that dying to self of which Christ is the exemplar and inspiration, and without which evil cannot be overcome.

3.24    When, however, this readiness to follow Christ is present, then God's purposes for human sexuality as a whole can begin to be discerned and enjoyed. This is true first for each individual. In thinking about

28

relationships we have already commented several times that these involve many different elements in our human nature, bodily, emotional, mental, spiritual, and so forth. For our health as human beings the whole of our self needs to be involved in whatever we are doing in the way appropriate to that particular situation. We are meant to live as a unity, not with one part of our self unacknowledged or at war with other parts. This need to be at unity within ourselves, to be what is commonly called an 'integrated' person, has two main implications. First, we are to grow to love every God-given aspect of our human nature – the capacity for prayer and worship, for thought and feeling, for physical activity of every kind, including the sexual. We are to love and value them all, even when they cannot be given full expression. But secondly, integration implies that all these elements in ourselves need to be in harmony, to co-operate. They cannot each go their own way. This means, as the wisdom of all ages has recognised, that some elements have to be subordinate to others. The raw energy of feeling or physical vitality must be harnessed and guided by the rational, ethical and spiritual self, if each of us is to become a unified moral person.

3.25    The hallowing and right direction of human sexuality also helps forward the redemption and sanctification of society. The way of chastity, whether in the married or unmarried state, followed as an offering in love to God and neighbour, is of great spiritual influence in changing values, lifting everyone's vision of what is both possible and of true worth, setting better standards of conduct, and healing the general sexual disorder and selfishness of the human race. In particular, where the obligation of chastity is accepted as the norm, the resultant security for individuals allows immensely more freedom in activities and relationships.

3.26    Lastly, the Christian vision for human sexuality looks beyond life in this world to its fulfilment in the world to come. In St Luke's Gospel words are ascribed to Jesus in reply to the Sadducees which have been influential in Christian thinking on this point: 'The men and women of this world marry; but those who have been judged worthy of a place in the other world, and of the resurrection from the dead, do not marry, for they are no longer subject to death. They are like angels; they are children of God, because they share in the resurrection' (Luke 20. 34-36, REB). Reflecting on these words today, we might want to say that our personhood is indissolubly bound up with our life-story as men or women, and that what that contributes can never be lost when our personal life is fulfilled in eternity. What will no longer be needed, as the passage makes clear, is the physical expression of sexuality, which is required now because of our mortality in order that human life may continue. By the same token this will liberate us to grow into the fullest possible relationship of love with all, being no longer restricted by the particularity of the flesh.

# 4.   The Phenomenon of Homosexual Love

4.1   In what follows we make frequent use, where helpful, of the term
'homophile', both the noun and the adjective, to refer to those who feel
erotic love for someone of the same sex. The word may have a somewhat
technical ring, but we have adopted it both because it is as yet free from
some of the negative overtones attaching to the term 'homosexual', and
because it can help to avoid clumsy circumlocutions in referring to
same-sex love.

4.2   It would be out of place here to attempt a full account of the
complex debate on the causes of homophile orientation, and of the
evidence for differing views. We most certainly wish, in agreement with
the Lambeth Conference resolution quoted earlier, to express our
support for further study and research, because the more truth, the more
light. But the situation at present is that experts are far from agreed on
answers. Some favour a physical explanation in terms of genetics or
biology, others a psychological, rooted in environment and upbringing.
Neither can yet be ruled out. There are statistics which hint at a hidden
genetic cause. There are also recurring psychological features in the
stories of homophiles which may be significant in a different direction.
Perhaps in many cases the truth will lie in a combination of both types of
cause. But even though the causality is as yet complex and unclear, one
may rightly warn against making improper use of possible explanations.
Some Christians, for example, have welcomed evidence for a genetic
origin as though it would confirm homosexuality as an alternative
condition within creation of equal validity with the heterosexual.
Similarly others have insisted on a psychological origin because this
would seem to offer better support for the belief that here we have a
distortion of the created order, not of God's making. In fact neither a
genetic nor a psychological explanation for a person's condition can itself
say whether a condition is good or bad, nor does a genetic origin mark a
particular condition as in accordance with the undistorted will of God.

4.3   In treating of homophile orientation we need to begin by
recognising its wide diversity. A great many human beings, indeed the
majority, at some stage in their lives, usually early adolescence, go
through a phase of homophile attraction. For most people this homophile
phase in their development soon passes, and is left behind for
heterosexual attachments, though in the opinion of many experts all

retain greater or lesser homophile elements in their personality, and can be placed, as it were, at a point on a spectrum. Some, however, never change to a dominant heterosexuality. Their homophile affections deepen and become their adult orientation. They feel no attraction to members of the opposite sex, and indeed may find such relationships intolerable. Yet others find themselves susceptible of strong attraction to both sexes. Finally we would note that while there are those who are comfortable with themselves only when they have accepted and affirmed their own homophile orientation, others find such acceptance impossible, and long for some way of escape.

4.4    This last point raises another issue, that namely of the possibility of changing a person's orientation. This subject is, understandably, highly sensitive in human terms. Some may wish for change, others find the very suggestion offensive. Here we would simply confine ourselves to a brief observation on what seem to be the clinical facts. First, no one can say as yet whether, if orientation is genetically controlled, it will one day be possible to modify it in a person's descendants. Secondly, if orientation is psychogenic, this does not necessarily mean that it can always be modified. Some people have experienced change as a result of a variety of approaches, either within psychotherapy or prayer counselling or a combination of both. Others have not changed but have been helped to be more whole and at peace in their situation. But the general verdict of those who work in this field is that sexual orientation, although it cannot be said without qualification to be fixed and final, is in most instances strongly resistant to modification. This would seem to be in keeping with the mystery of its causation, a mystery reflected in the diversity of theories on the subject. Nevertheless it would be wise to ponder one point in good time. If research does eventually show that a homophile orientation is genetic in origin, and if it then becomes possible to eliminate that orientation in future generations by genetic engineering, what will be the ethical criteria for deciding whether or not such a change should be made?

4.5    The general tendency in public discussion is to concentrate on the differences, real or alleged, between heterophiles and homophiles. We regard it as of the first importance to take the opposite line, and to emphasise the common humanity which they share. It ought not to need stating, but it still does, that the same range of talents, virtues, vices, interests and aptitudes is found in both. When talking of homophiles and heterophiles, we are speaking of fellow human beings whose contributions to the life of us all are, whether for good or ill, in overwhelming degree alike.

4.6    It is of equal importance to recognise the common ground in their emotional experiences. Both speak of the attraction which is called 'falling in love', and which gives the beloved that special quality and value that sets them apart from all others. Both know the longing for an exclusively close relationship with the other person, the need to spend as much time as possible and to share as much as possible of one's life with them, and the desire to express one's affection and commitment by mutual physical enjoyment and self-giving. Likewise among both homophiles and heterophiles there is the same variation in the degree to which the ideal of a loving relationship is achieved. Among both there are the shallow, the immature, the inconstant, the selfish and the cruel. There are the promiscuous, those interested only in physical satisfaction, and those seemingly incapable of commitment and loyalty at any level of the personality. But equally among both there are those who grow steadily in fidelity and in mutual caring, understanding and support, whose partnerships are a blessing to the world around them, and who achieve great, even heroic sacrifice and devotion.

4.7    We need also to be alive to the question of the social network within which all individuals have to make their way. Again it is as true for homophiles as for heterophiles that personal relationships need a supporting community, a social environment with conventions and expectations which largely determine the character and significance of such relationships, and which give those involved in them a broad code of behaviour toward their partner and toward outsiders. At the simplest human level most of us need and want to be free to share some of our experience with others, to talk about the things most precious to us, or at any rate to move among friends and neighbours who understand and accept what we are trying to do with our lives. All this is as true for the homophile as for the heterophile. But because society at large finds it hard to understand or to affirm the homophile as a person, these needs are not ordinarily met. The result is the formation of exclusive social groupings in which the homophile can feel at home without explanation or reserve. We would hope that such groupings would not be the only social environment available for the homophile. With regard to the Church in particular, we would draw attention to the need for congregations to be places of open acceptance and friendship for homophiles as for people of every kind, both generally and in such settings as the best sort of house group.

4.8   We recognise that there are major questions to be faced concerning the attitudes to homophiles in both Church and society. The phenomenon of homophobia is very real, and is not confined to those who actively persecute homosexuals. Repugnance at homophile behaviour (actual or imagined) and fear of the danger to others from tolerating or seeming to encourage it can combine even in the reasonable and charitable to foster underlying feelings of hostility toward gay and lesbian people. The effects of such attitudes, both overt and covert, are twofold. One effect is to drive some homophiles underground. This inevitably makes it more difficult for them to build lasting relationships, and increases the temptations to infidelity and promiscuity. In addition the untruths and concealment to which some homophiles are driven for self-protection, and the constant fear that others will sooner or later penetrate the facade behind which much of their life has to be conducted, are corrosive of personal integrity. By contrast other homophiles, who refuse to be trapped in these ways, are driven to protest by taking up a defiant stance, demonstrating their pride in being gay or lesbian, and making exaggerated claims and demands. This further polarises what is already a situation of conflict, and leads others who were sympathetic to be hostile. The complexity of the situation, however, should not blind us to the clear, simple and fundamental responsibility of Christians to reject and resist all forms of homophobia. This carries with it the duty to be active in protecting those who are victimised, since it is sadly true that members of the gay and lesbian community are all too often not only verbally disparaged and abused or made the targets of cruel so-called 'humour', but are also physically assaulted.

4.9   There are, as one might expect, misconceptions among many heterosexual people as to the ways in which homophiles, male or female, give their love physical expression. It is not our intention to enter into detail on this matter here. Brief clinical descriptions say nothing about the human reality of either homosexual or heterosexual love-making. What perhaps should be said is that the greater part of the repertory of both kinds of physical love is the same; and that where in either case this involves clinical abuse of the human body that is to be deplored.

4.10   For both heterophile and homophile the genital organs are the key to a full physical expression of love. Moreover, because they are universally regarded as the most private area of the body, contact with those of another person is a uniquely intimate act. When a relationship admits of such contact, therefore, it has (or ought to have) moved on to a new level of personal commitment. Hence the stress laid in statements such as the motion passed by General Synod in 1987 on what are called 'genital acts'. The distinction thus drawn has been questioned, but it would seem to be valid. It is true, of course, that there is a continuum of physical manifestations of erotic feeling from first attraction to full arousal, and that genital pleasure may play its part in this from an early stage. But deliberate genital contact does nevertheless represent the crossing of a significant boundary.

4.11   By bearing this distinction in mind it is possible also to say something which we believe may be helpful about Christ's teaching in Matthew 5.27-28, characterising looking lustfully on a woman as 'adultery in the heart'. As we are sexual beings, erotic feelings will spontaneously arise at the sight of someone who attracts us in that way. A healthy spirituality will not deplore this as a sign of depravity. The sin against which Jesus warns is pursuing in fantasy the fulfilment of some action which in real life would be a sin. Where, however, a Christian's spontaneous feelings are homophile, he or she may be troubled by the anxiety that any imagination, even the feeling itself, is sinful. In our view this is not what Christ meant, and is humanly destructive as causing the person concerned to regard himself or herself as evil in the very substance of their being, which is absolutely not the case.

4.12   We turn now to a question which has been fundamental in Christian discussions of sexuality. It has been a theme of Christian tradition, ever since St Paul's words in the first chapter of Romans, to classify certain sexual activities and practices, those of homophiles most particularly, as unnatural or contrary to nature. In recent years this categorisation has been fiercely contested by those who argue that same-sex love is simply one legitimate way of being human within the wide diversity of God's created order, and should be accepted as such and affirmed as of equal validity with the heterosexual.

4.13   We believe it is important to give careful thought to this issue. The word 'natural' has various connotations. Like many other words it takes its meaning in a particular context from some implied contrast. Plants, animals, landscapes may be natural by contrast with what is man-made. A spontaneous personal manner is called natural by contrast with one which is studied or artificial. Some skill or ability may be natural as opposed to one acquired by study and practice. Again 'natural' may be used in contrast to 'cultural'; or in theology 'natural' may refer to what can be concluded about God by unaided reasoning from experience of the created order, as distinct from 'revealed' theology whose truths are communicated by divine inspiration or action. By extension from this last use of 'natural', moral theology employs it to describe those types of human conduct which are in harmony with the will of God as discernible from creation as opposed to those which violate that will and which are 'unnatural'. In this context, therefore, 'natural' does not refer simply to whatever we happen to find human beings doing or wanting to do spontaneously. Thus we can say that, though in certain circumstances it may, in ordinary parlance, be a very natural thing to tell a lie, in the theological sense it will be 'unnatural', because if God created a world in which accurate communication is possible we may properly assume that his overall purpose was to enable us to give and receive the truth. But it may not always be unnatural in this sense to lie, as in the classic example of lying to divert a murderer from his intended victim, where the lie serves God's overriding purposes of love and justice.

4.14    In the context of human sexuality, a first and obvious observation is that sexual desire and the sexual activity that results from it serve the purposes of procreation; and it would be highly unreasonable to argue that it was not the will of a Creator that this should be so. Furthermore, since it is the interaction of the male and female genital organs which makes procreation possible, that too must be part of God's purpose, and be so for at least the great majority of humankind. In short the biological evidence is at least compatible with a theological view that heterosexual physical union is divinely intended to be the norm.

4.15    At the same time such sexual desire and intercourse have other, if related consequences, of which the availability of effective contraceptive methods has increased the importance. The intimacy of the parents, and the pleasure they find in each other, serve to strengthen the bond between them and so to enhance their co-operation in the necessary work of raising and protecting their children and bringing them to mature adulthood. But if that is the practical utility of sexual affection, it can also help to create the same kind of bond whether there are children or not. The words of Genesis about the union of man and woman are true independently of procreation. Adam amid all the richness of creation finds himself in lonely isolation; among all other creatures there is 'no helper fit for him'. In the story only the creation of another who is bone of his bone and flesh of his flesh overcomes this loneliness; and, as the text observes, this is the fundamental reason why 'a man leaves his father and mother and attaches himself to his wife, and the two become one' (Gen.2.24, REB).

4.16   The potential blessings of this bonding are such that a theology of creation will very properly see them as also 'natural', that is, within the purposes of God. Moreover these blessings are not simply there to be received automatically. They depend very greatly on the willingness of partners to give themselves to one another. This is true of the physical relationship, which is never all it can be if either simply takes with no thought of giving – a reflection which is by no means as modern as it sounds, but is found in writers of the ancient classical world. But the pattern of self-giving needed for physical fulfilment is also essential if the partnership is to realise its full potential in other ways. In this way physical sex can positively promote personal values which Christians will certainly see as very much God's will for human life.

4.17   In heterosexual love this personal bonding and mutual self-giving happen between two people who, because they are of different gender, are not merely physically differentiated but also diverse in their emotional, mental and spiritual lives, their way of experiencing and responding to reality. It is important not to exaggerate this distinction. As the writer of Genesis 2 realised, the fact of the common humanity of women and men is more important than any differences between them. Nevertheless they do live that common humanity in different ways which make the distinctive contributions of each essential for the fullness of humankind as a whole; and it is important for the mature development both of individual men and women and of society that each person should come to understand and to value this complementarity. The place where people normally begin to do this is the family, headed by a father and a mother, before going on to their own wider experience in society, marriage and parenthood. These structures have not always served the growth of true complementarity in the way they ought to have done, for they have too often denied women their full place and potential, and thus also denied men the experience of human life as God means it to be. The remedy, however, is not to attempt the impossible task of replacing structures which are deeply embedded in the fundamental order of creation, but to inspire them with true values and to use them for right purposes. The fact that heterosexual unions in the context of marriage and the family are of such primary importance for the fostering of true man-woman complementarity seems to us to confirm their essential place in God's providential order.

4.18    These considerations suggest one further insight. If the physical differentiation between the sexes is not only relevant to the biological process of reproduction but is also integral to the personal spiritual realities of mutual self-giving, parenthood and complementarity, then this is a major instance of a principle that lies at the heart of the Christian world-view: that the physical order is sacramental. We have spoken earlier of the intimate union and mutual dependence of the bodily and the spiritual in the biblical understanding of humanity. Through that union the physical life of the person can both express inner spiritual realities and nourish their development. The very phrase 'to make love', if used with true understanding, would catch this inter-relation exactly. Our bodies can be the means of forwarding a spiritual and, where there is a living relationship with God, a divine purpose in our lives. For this to happen, however, there has to be a harmony between the physical and the spiritual. When we think of our bodies in this light, we see that they need to be used in a way that is both proper to themselves and in harmony with the spiritual realities we are trying to express and foster. Psychologically this corresponds to the ideal of an integrated human personality, where body, feelings, mind and spirit work fully together. Theologically it corresponds to the desire that every aspect of ourselves should be aligned with God's will.

4.19    In the area of sexuality as in all others everyone, both homophile and heterophile, falls short of whole and integrated personal being, either through limitations and distortions in themselves or through force of circumstances. What is 'natural' theologically is certainly not 'natural' for all men and women in the everyday sense of that word. Everything has to be redeemed. Nevertheless those who are homophile can find themselves faced with specific difficulties distinct from those of the majority. There is, for example, a mismatch between their sexuality and their physical and often also their emotional capacity for parenthood.

There may be for some a mismatch between their bodies and the ways in which they wish to express their mutual self-giving. Their sexuality can be a barrier rather than a help toward full man-woman complementarity. In all these respects, therefore, there are special difficulties in the way of integrating their sexuality into their life as a whole, or of fulfilling its potential as a sacramental expression of their relationship with the one they love. The task that surely faces both the individual Christian homophile and the Church is to work out together how his or her sexuality can best find expression within the discipleship to which every human being is called.

# 5.  The Homosexual in the Life and Fellowship of the Church

5.1   We come now to consider what guidance for pastoral practice can be offered to the Church in the present state of Christian understanding of this issue. The aim of us all must be to allow the Holy Spirit to lead us into the mind of Christ for all his members in a world where homosexual orientation is the experience of some. We begin by setting out two fundamental principles of equal validity and significance.

5.2   The first is that homophile orientation and its expression in sexual activity do not constitute a parallel and alternative form of human sexuality as complete within the terms of the created order as the heterosexual. The convergence of Scripture, Tradition and reasoned reflection on experience, even including the newly sympathetic and perceptive thinking of our own day, make it impossible for the Church to come with integrity to any other conclusion. Heterosexuality and homosexuality are not equally congruous with the observed order of creation or with the insights of revelation as the Church engages with these in the light of her pastoral ministry.

5.3   We are aware that some regard such a position as tantamount to a rejection of the homophile as a person. Personal identity, it is argued, is so fundamentally bound up with sexuality that to categorise the latter as in some way imperfect is to treat the whole person as also essentially inferior. The argument is, however, false. Sexuality is a very important and influential element in our human make-up, but it is only one aspect of it. Our sexuality may vary from the norm in many ways, of which a homophile orientation is but one, without affecting our equal worth and dignity as human beings, which rests on the fact that all of us alike are made in the image of God. It is crucial to stress this point, because by equating the principle set out in the preceding paragraph with an inhuman rejection of the homophile person great harm has been done. Sexuality is given an inflated significance in human life; homophiles are wrongly made to feel devalued by the traditional teaching of the Church; and those who hold to that teaching are pressed to abandon it by implied accusations of cruelty and injustice.

5.4   This leads directly to our second fundamental principle, laid upon us by the truths at the very heart of the faith: homosexual people are in every way as valuable to and as valued by God as heterosexual people. God loves us all alike, and has for each one of us a range of possibilities within his design for the universe. This includes those who, for whatever reason, find themselves with a homophile orientation which, so far as anyone at present can tell, cannot in their case be changed, and within which therefore they have the responsibility of living human life creatively and well. Every human being has a unique potential for Christlikeness, and an individual contribution to make through that likeness to the final consummation of all things.

5.5   Of Christian homophiles some are clear that the way they must follow to fulfil this calling is to witness to God's general will for human sexuality by a life of abstinence. In the power of the Holy Spirit and out of love for Christ they embrace the self-denial involved, gladly and trustfully opening themselves to the power of God's grace to order and fulfil their personalities within this way of life. This is a path of great faithfulness, travelled often under the weight of a very heavy cross. It is deserving of all praise and of the support of Church members through prayer, understanding and active friendship.

5.6   At the same time there are others who are conscientiously convinced that this way of abstinence is not the best for them, and that they have more hope of growing in love for God and neighbour with the help of a loving and faithful homophile partnership, in intention lifelong, where mutual self-giving includes the physical expression of their attachment. In responding to this conviction it is important to bear in mind the historic tension in Christian ethical thinking between the God-given moral order and the freedom of the moral agent. While insisting that conscience needs to be informed in the light of that order, Christian tradition also contains an emphasis on respect for free conscientious judgement where the individual has seriously weighed the issues involved. The homophile is only one in a range of such cases. While unable, therefore, to commend the way of life just described as in itself as faithful a reflection of God's purposes in creation as the heterophile, we do not reject those who sincerely believe it is God's call to them. We stand alongside them in the fellowship of the Church, all alike dependent upon the undeserved grace of God. All those who seek to live their lives in Christ owe one another friendship and understanding. It is therefore important that in every congregation such homophiles should find fellow-Christians who will sensitively and naturally provide this for them. Indeed, if this is not done, any professions on the part of the Church that it is committed to openness and learning about the homophile situation can be no more than empty words.

5.7   It will be noted that what we have said no more countenances promiscuous, casual or exploitative sex for the homophile than for the heterophile. The ideal of chastity holds good for all Christians; and homophiles who do not renounce all physical sex relations must nevertheless be guided by some form of that ideal appropriate to them. In this regard we would make specific comments on three particular matters, all connected in some way with the themes of fidelity and the personal dimension in sexual relations.

5.8   The first is that of bisexuality. We recognise that there are those whose sexual orientation is ambiguous, and who can find themselves attracted to partners of either sex. Nevertheless it is clear that bisexual activity must always be wrong for this reason, if for no other, that it inevitably involves being unfaithful. The Church's guidance to bisexual Christians is that if they are capable of heterophile relationships and of satisfaction within them, they should follow the way of holiness in either celibacy or abstinence or heterosexual marriage. In the situation of the bisexual it can also be that counselling will help the person concerned to discover the truth of their personality and to achieve a degree of inner healing.

5.9   The second concern arises from developments in the ideology of homosexual relations. The argument is heard that the norm of a faithful one-to-one relationship – dismissed as 'coupledom' – is simply an alien legacy from the heterophile world with its family and social responsibilities. By contrast the homophile can and should enjoy the freedom to express through physical sex a whole range of relationships, profound or superficial, transient or longer lasting, with any number of partners. Clearly this flies in the face of all that has been said earlier about the sacramentality of the body and the importance of proportion between physical intimacy and personal commitment. It should, indeed, be recognised that one-to-one partnerships are not the only ethically serious model for homophiles, who may find that the more appropriate way of life for them is, for example, that of à network of warmly, even intensely emotional friendships. But the attack on permanent partnerships here described has nothing to do with such alternatives, but is simply a pretentious disguise for the evil of promiscuity. Its emergence, we believe, should make Christians more aware of the importance of faithfulness and commitment in relationships.

5.10   The third matter is that of paedophilia. This may be either homosexual or heterosexual. Because, however, it is commonly linked in popular misconception with homosexuality, let it be stated yet again that a homophile orientation does not, any more than a heterophile, of itself entail a sexual interest in or attraction to children. It is mistaken and unjust to assume, for example, that children in school or in a church choir are particularly at risk from gay or lesbian members of staff. Turning to the question of paedophilia itself, those who promote or practise it often claim that sexual activity expresses and enhances a personal relationship between adult and child. This claim is to be totally rejected. Whatever the paedophile may choose to believe, a child is not capable of integrating physical sexual activity into a genuinely personal relationship, nor can there be that equality and complementarity between an adult and a child which is proper to sexual relations. Inevitably, therefore, paedophilia becomes abuse by the adult of the child, with all the damage and distortion to the child's personality which that entails. Paedophilia breaches the limits of what is right and healthy in the child–adult relationship, and in Christian terms is a sin not only against chastity but also against charity and justice. To these evils paedophilia adds the further danger of making it difficult later for the child to achieve a mature adult sexuality.

5.11   We come now to the question of the homophile clergy. Within the population as a whole a small percentage is predominantly homophile in orientation. It may well be that in the ordained ministry, as in the arts and the caring professions, the percentage is higher. We believe that the great majority of such clergy are not in sexually active partnerships. What we know for a fact is that the ministries of many homophile clergy are highly dedicated and have been greatly blessed. God has endowed them with spiritual gifts, as he has his other ministers, and we give thanks for all alike.

5.12   There are, however, questions to be faced concerning the ministry of homophile clergy who believe that the right way of life for them is that of an exclusive and permanent but also sexually active partnership. These questions are additional to those which arise in the case of the Christian people in general, and they relate to the representative and pastoral responsibilities of the clergy.

5.13    From the time of the New Testament onwards it has been expected of those appointed to the ministry of authority in the Church that they shall not only preach but also live the Gospel. These expectations are as real today as ever they were. People not only inside the Church but outside it believe rightly that in the way of life of an ordained minister they ought to be able to see a pattern which the Church commends. Inevitably, therefore, the world will assume that all ways of living which an ordained person is allowed to adopt are in Christian eyes equally valid. With regard to homophile relationships, however, this is, as we have already explained, a position which for theological reasons the Church does not hold. Justice does indeed demand that the Church should be free in its pastoral discretion to accommodate a God-given ideal to human need, so that individuals are not turned away from God and their neighbour but helped to grow in love toward both from within their own situation. But the Church is also bound to take care that the ideal itself is not misrepresented or obscured; and to this end the example of its ordained ministers is of crucial significance. This means that certain possibilities are not open to the clergy by comparison with the laity, something that in principle has always been accepted.

5.14    Restrictions on what the clergy may do also stem from their pastoral function. If they are to be accessible and acceptable to the greatest number of people, both within the Church and outside it, then so far as possible their lives must be free of anything which will make it difficult for others to have confidence in them as messengers, watchmen and stewards of the Lord. There can be no doubt that an ordained person living in an active homophile relationship does for a significant number of people at this time present such a difficulty.

5.15    Some would argue that a deeper understanding of God's will would show these difficulties to be unfounded. The Church, they would say, needs to undergo a profound and radical transformation of its attitude to and understanding of the whole of human sexuality, including homophile relationships. Homophile couples, on this view, are simply witnessing to part of a truth which the Church will eventually come to accept, and ought to be allowed freedom for that witness. To this we would reply that, though the Church is not infallible, there is at any given time such a thing as the mind of the Church on matters of faith and life. Those who disagree with that mind are free to argue for change. What they are not free to do is to go against that mind in their own practice.

5.16   Another dissenting view is that clergy living in such permanent and faithful relationships are needed in order to provide others in the same situation both with role models and with wise and understanding pastoral care. On the question of the clergy as role models, the Ordinal of 1662 and the Canon Law do indeed require those ordained deacon and priest to make both themselves and their families wholesome examples and patterns to the flock of Christ. But this points to a particular difficulty as regards clergy in sexually active homophile partnerships, namely that, given the present understanding of such partnerships in the Church as a whole, it is unrealistic to suppose that these clergy could in most parishes be accepted as examples to the whole flock as distinct from the homophiles within it. On the second point, that of good pastoral care, it is mistaken to suggest that this can be given only by those who have shared the relevant experience. Shared experience can in some cases enhance pastoral care, but if it were essential no pastors would be able to help or guide more than a small proportion of those to whom they were called to minister. The good pastor who, in the power of the Holy Spirit, looks honestly into his or her own heart, and is prepared to listen and observe sensitively and imaginatively, will have sufficient empathy to be able to bring the Gospel truth-in-love to bear in word and deed. Finally on this question, we would point out that in a mature Christian congregation pastoral care for distinctive needs of any kind does not all have to be provided by the clergy alone.

5.17   We have, therefore, to say that in our considered judgement the clergy cannot claim the liberty to enter into sexually active homophile relationships. Because of the distinctive nature of their calling, status and consecration, to allow such a claim on their part would be seen as placing that way of life in all respects on a par with heterosexual marriage as a reflection of God's purposes in creation. The Church cannot accept such a parity and remain faithful to the insights which God has given it through Scripture, tradition and reasoned reflection on experience.

5.18   In the light of this judgement some may propose that bishops should be more rigorous in searching out and exposing clergy who may be in sexually active homophile relationships. We reject this approach for two reasons. First, there is a growing tendency today to regard any two people of the same sex who choose to make their home together as being in some form of erotic relationship. This is a grossly unfair assumption, which can give rise to much unhappiness, and the Church should do nothing that might seem to countenance or promote it. Secondly, it has always been the practice of the Church of England to trust its members, and not to carry out intrusive interrogations in order to make sure that they are behaving themselves. Any general inquisition into the conduct of the clergy would not only infringe their right to privacy but would manifest a distrust not consonant with the commission entrusted to them, and likely to undermine their confidence and morale. Although we must take steps to avoid public scandal and to protect the Church's teaching, we shall continue, as we have done hitherto, to treat all clergy who give no occasion for scandal with trust and respect, and we expect all our fellow Christians to do the same.

5.19   This, however, leaves unanswered the question of those clergy who feel it their duty to come out, that is, to make known publicly either their orientation or their practice. Within this group there are two main categories. The first ought to present no problem to anyone. It consists simply of those who wish it to be known that they are homophile in orientation, but who are committed to a life of abstinence. Their desire is to be free to live among their neighbours with dignity and without concealment, unembarrassed, for example, by speculation or by suggestions of marriage. A community which cannot accept such an honourable candour is not worthy of the name of Christian. We greatly regret the way in which candidates for appointment who are open in this way are often rejected by parishes and others solely on these grounds.

5.20   The second category comprises those who are themselves in active homophile partnerships, and who come out as a matter of personal integrity. They believe their relationship to be right in the sight of God, and find concealment both repugnant and destructive; or they feel it their duty to show solidarity with others in the same situation. Inevitably such a declaration is also in effect a pre-emptive action within the movement for change in the Church's perceptions and teaching on this whole question, and therefore raises the issue we have already identified in 5.15 above.

5.21   We respect that integrity. But it is also our duty to affirm the whole pattern of Christian teaching on sexuality set out in these pages, and to uphold those requirements for conduct which will best witness to it. We therefore call upon all clergy to live lives that respect the Church's teaching, and we shall do everything in our power to help them to do so.

5.22   This means that candidates for ordination also must be prepared to abide by the same standards. For reasons already mentioned, however, we do not think it right to interrogate individuals on their sexual lives, unless there are strong reasons for doing so. Ordinarily it should be left to candidates' own consciences to act responsibly in this matter.

5.23   Let us try to sum up the essential points of the guidance we are seeking to give in this chapter. The Church in its pastoral mission ought to help and encourage all its members, as they pursue their pilgrimage from the starting-points given in their own personalities and circumstances, and as they grow by grace within their own particular potential. It is, therefore, only right that there should be an open and welcoming place in the Christian community both for those homophiles who follow the way of abstinence, giving themselves to friendship for many rather than to intimacy with one, and also for those who are conscientiously convinced that a faithful, sexually active relationship with one other person, aimed at helping both partners to grow in discipleship, is the way of life God wills for them. But the Church exists also to live out in the world the truth it has been given about the nature of God's creation, the way of redemption through the Cross, and the ultimate hope of newness and fullness of life. We have judged that we ourselves and all clergy, as consecrated public and representative figures, entrusted with the message and means of grace, have a responsibility on behalf of the whole Body of Christ to show the primacy of this truth by striving to embody it in our own lives. But we also wish to stress the Church's care for and value of all her clergy alike, and that where the Church's teaching results for any ordained person in a burden grievous to be borne we, the bishops, as pastors to the pastors, will always be ready to share in any way we can in the bearing of that burden.

5.24   In conclusion we return to the observation quoted in our opening chapter concerning the many fundamental questions which underlie this whole debate. The predicament of the conscientious Christian homophile raises complex issues. How are we to use the Scriptures to guide us today? What is the relation between law and grace for a Christian who seeks to follow Christ in the freedom of the Spirit? Granted that we all have to start our Christian pilgrimage from where we are, how diverse can the journeys be by which we come home to God? Given the complex tangle of human sexuality, and the fact that sexuality as such may have no place in eternal life, is specific sexual conduct as important for our destiny as the values and attitudes expressed through it? On what understanding of the ordained ministry do we base our requirements of different standards for the clergy and the laity, and are we coherent or consistent in these demands? These are the kind of questions to which we have had to reply with practical guidance for our Church in this particular time, society and culture. In making our response we have tried never to forget our two principal duties as bishops: to be guardians of the Christian faith and way of life; yet equally to be pastors who not only respond in love to those who cry out of any pain of injustice or distress but also seek to discern when love is summoning the Church to rethink its existing perception of the truth. The story of the Church's attitude to homosexuals has too often been one of prejudice, ignorance and oppression. All of us need to acknowledge that, and to repent for any part we may have had in it. The Church has begun to listen to its homophile brothers and sisters, and must deepen and extend that listening, finding through joint prayer and reflection a truer understanding and the love that casts out fear. If we are faithful to Our Lord, then disagreement over the proper expression of homosexual love will never become rejection of the homosexual person.